Made in the USA
Columbia, SC
25 January 2024

30862905R00059